How to Make Ubtan Powder

Dr Miriam Kinai

Copyright © 2013 Dr Miriam Kinai

http://thebestsellingebooks.blogspot.com/

All rights reserved. No part of this publication may be reproduced or transmitted in any form or by any means, electronic or mechanical, including photocopying, recording, or by any information storage and retrieval system, without written permission from the author, except for the inclusion of brief quotations in a review.

ISBN: 1482570440

ISBN-13: 978-1482570441

Contents

1	What is Ubtan Powder?	Pg #1
2	Ubtan Powder Ingredients	Pg #2
3	Bridal Ubtan Powder Recipe	Pg #11
4	How to Modify Ubtan Powder Recipes for: Normal skin, Sensitive skin, Dry skin, Mature skin, Prematurely aging skin, Cellulite	Pg #13
5	Characteristics of the following Essential Oils: Clary sage, Eucalyptus, Geranium, Grapefruit, Lavender, Lemon, Lemongrass, Roman chamomile, Spearmint, Sweet orange, Rosemary, Peppermint, Tea tree, Ylang ylang	Pg #21

Dr. Miriam Kinai

1
What Is Ubtan Powder?

Ubtans are traditional Indians masks which are used to cleanse the skin, exfoliate it, nourish and protect it.

Ubtans were and are still used before weddings by brides and grooms since they help the skin glow with radiant beauty and health. They can be applied either on the whole body or just on the face.

*****

2
Ubtan Powder Ingredients

Ubtan recipes vary from source to source and the following are some of the ingredients commonly used to make them:

1. Sandalwood Powder

Sandalwood powder has the following health benefits and uses:

1. Managing oily skin to prevent acne lesions.

2. Managing dry skin conditions with cracked and chapped skin.

3. Managing sensitive skin.

4. Management of prematurely aging and mature skin.

5. Has antiseptic properties and helps cuts and burns heal.

6. Useful for scars and stretch marks.

7. Mentally calming and used to manage stress and nervous tension.

8. Cheering and useful for relieving feelings of sadness.

9. It is also said to have aphrodisiac properties.

2. Rose Powder

Rose powder has the following health benefits and uses due to its numerous properties:

1. Useful for all skin types including dry, oily, sensitive, mature and prematurely aging skin.

2. Astringent properties that help regulate the skin's oil production without drying it and thus useful for oily and acne prone skin.

3. Skin soothing properties and thus useful for sensitive skin types.

4. Hydrating properties and thus useful for dry skin types and mature skin.

5. Anti-inflammatory properties and thus useful for conditions like eczema.

6. Anti-septic properties and immune stimulant properties and useful for skin infections.

7. Exfoliates and tones the skin giving it a great glow.

8. Mentally calming properties and used for stress management, post traumatic shock disorder (PTSD), anxiety, anger management and to relieve tension headaches and nervous tension.

9. Cheering and balancing properties and used for depression, post partum depression, sorrow and heartache.

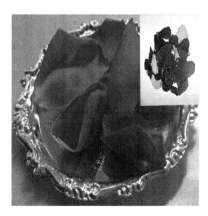

3. Cosmetic Clays

Cosmetic clays are rich in minerals and they cleanse and exfoliate the skin as well as stimulate its circulation.

Different clays are used for different skin types for example:

Normal skin types can use rose clay, yellow kaolin clay.

Dry skin types can use rose clay, white kaolin clay, yellow kaolin clay, Moroccan red clay.

Oily skin types can use Bentonite clay, French green clay, multani mitti clay, rhassoul clay, glacial clay.

Sensitive skin types can use white kaolin clay, yellow kaolin clay.

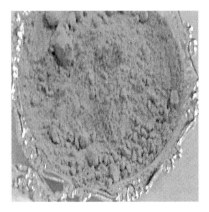

***

4. Almond Powder

Almond powder or almond meal contains essential fatty acids and vitamins. It therefore nourishes and softens the skin while getting rid of the dead cells on the skin's surface.

Almond flour is also useful for unclogging skin pores since it absorbs excess oil from the skin.

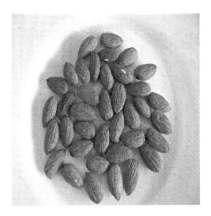

***

5. Turmeric

Turmeric has the following uses due to its numerous properties:

1. Antibacterial, antiviral and antifungal properties and is therefore useful for preventing skin infections.

2. Antiseptic properties are also useful for the management of acne.

3. Anti-inflammatory properties and has been shown to reduce the inflammation associated with psoriasis.

4. Has antioxidants which provide protection against free radical cell damage.

5. Turmeric may also speed up wound healing due to its anti-oxidant and anti-inflammatory effects.

6. It is also used in the management of dry skin conditions.

7. It is also used to manage mature skin since it reduces the appearance of wrinkles.

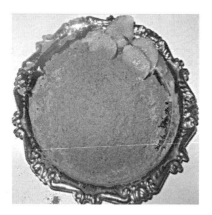

***

8. Gram Flour

Gram flour is made by grinding chickpeas. It is also known as chickpea flour or besan. It cleanses the skin and exfoliates it.

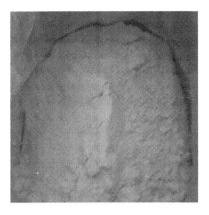

***

9. Rice Flour

Rice flour is made by grinding rice. It is suitable for all skin types from dry to oily, sensitive and mature.

It cleanses the skin and exfoliates it leaving it brighter and glowing without shining since it absorbs excess oil.

Rice flour is also said to have anti-aging properties and is used to prevent premature aging of the skin. It is thought to increase collagen production by the skin since its chemical structure is similar to that of ceramide.

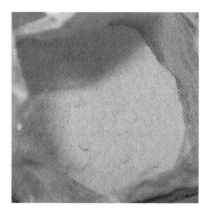

***

10. Yogurt

Yogurt helps remove the dead cells from the skin's surface and reveal the youthful skin beneath them since it contains lactic acid. It also hydrates the skin.

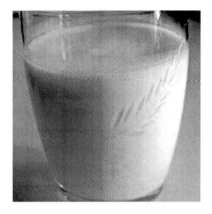

* * * * *

3
Bridal Ubtan Powder Recipe

Ingredients

2 tablespoons rice flour

2 tablespoons sandalwood powder

2 tablespoons almond powder

2 tablespoons rose petal powder

2 tablespoons cosmetic clay

2 tablespoons turmeric powder

2 tablespoons gram flour

½ cup Yogurt

Instructions

Mix all the dry ingredients together and store in an airtight container.

To use, mix 4 tablespoons of the dry mixture with 2 tablespoons of yogurt to form a thick paste.

Apply the mixture as you massage it over the entire body and let it dry.

Rinse it off with warm water.

Moisturize the skin.

Repeat for 40 days before your wedding day if you want soft, glowing skin on your big day.

Tips

1. Traditionally, brides were massaged with sesame oil before the ubtan was applied and you can also do it this way.

2. Use the correct cosmetic clay for your skin type. See chapter 1

3. If you do not have sandalwood powder, you can add 3 drops of sandalwood essential oil instead.

4. If you do not have rose powder, you can add 3 drops of rose essential oil instead.

5. If you do not have almond powder, you can add 2 tablespoons of sweet almond oil instead.

* * * * *

4
How To Modify Ubtan Powder Recipes

Ingredients

2 tablespoons rice flour

2 tablespoons sandalwood powder

2 tablespoons almond powder

2 tablespoons rose petal powder

2 tablespoons cosmetic clay

2 tablespoons turmeric powder

2 tablespoons gram flour

The above basic bridal ubtan recipe can be modified to suit different skin types in the following way:

1. By using different liquids to prepare it

2. By adding different essential oils

USING DIFFERENT LIQUIDS

The basic bridal ubtan powder recipe can be modified for different skin types by using various liquid mediums like egg whites, egg yolks, aloe vera gel, yogurt, butter milk, whole milk, heavy cream, coconut milk, wheatgerm oil, almond oil, lemon juice or water.

1. Oily Skin Ubtan Recipe

Mix all the dry bridal ubtan recipe ingredients together and store in an airtight container.

To use, mix 2 tablespoons of the dry mixture with one egg white or one tablespoon of aloe vera gel or yogurt or butter milk or water.

Apply the mixture as you massage it over the entire body and let it dry.

Rinse it off with warm water.

Moisturize the skin.

* * *

2. Dry Skin and Mature Skin Ubtan Recipe

Mix all the dry bridal ubtan recipe ingredients together and store in an airtight container.

To use, mix 2 tablespoons of the dry mixture with one egg yolk or one tablespoon of whole cow's milk or heavy cream or yogurt or coconut milk or wheatgerm oil.

Apply the mixture as you massage it over the entire body and let it dry.

Rinse it off with warm water.

Moisturize the skin.

* * *

3. Combination Skin Ubtan Recipe

Mix all the dry bridal ubtan recipe ingredients together and store in an airtight container.

To use, mix 2 tablespoons of the dry mixture with one whole egg or one tablespoon of almond oil or aloe vera juice or lemon juice.

Apply the mixture as you massage it over the entire body and let it dry.

Rinse it off with warm water.

Moisturize the skin.

* * * *

USING DIFFERENT ESSENTIAL OILS

The basic bridal ubtan powder recipe can be modified for different skin types by using various essential oils. For example

1. Normal Skin Ubtan Powder Recipe

Mix all the dry bridal ubtan recipe ingredients together and store in an airtight container.

To use, mix 2 tablespoons of the dry mixture with one egg or one tablespoon of whole cow's milk or yogurt or coconut milk.

Add 10 drops of essential oils that are beneficial for normal skin like clary sage, roman chamomile, eucalyptus, geranium, rosemary, tea tree, lavender, lemon, peppermint, and ylang ylang essential oils.

Apply the mixture as you massage it over the entire body and let it dry.

Rinse it off with warm water.

Moisturize the skin.

* * *

2. Oily Skin Ubtan Recipe

Mix all the dry bridal ubtan recipe ingredients together and store in an airtight container.

To use, mix 2 tablespoons of the dry mixture with one egg white or one tablespoon of aloe vera gel or yogurt or butter milk or water.

Add 10 drops of essential oils that are beneficial for oily skin like tea tree, lavender, and lemon essential oils.

Apply the mixture as you massage it over the entire body and let it dry.

Rinse it off with warm water.

Moisturize the skin.

3. Combination Skin Ubtan Recipe

Mix all the dry bridal ubtan recipe ingredients together and store in an airtight container.

To use, mix 2 tablespoons of the dry mixture with one whole egg or one tablespoon of almond oil or aloe vera juice or lemon juice.

Add 10 drops of essential oils that are beneficial for combination skin like tea tree and lavender essential oils.

Apply the mixture as you massage it over the entire body and let it dry.

Rinse it off with warm water.

Moisturize the skin.

* * *

4. Dry Skin Ubtan Recipe

Mix all the dry bridal ubtan recipe ingredients together and store in an airtight container.

To use, mix 2 tablespoons of the dry mixture with one egg yolk or one tablespoon of whole cow's milk or heavy cream or yogurt or coconut milk or wheatgerm oil.

Add 10 drops of essential oils used to manage dry skin like lavender, Roman chamomile, and ylang ylang.

Apply the mixture as you massage it over the entire body and let it dry.

Rinse it off with warm water.

Moisturize the skin.

* * *

5. Mature Skin Ubtan Recipe

Mix all the dry bridal ubtan recipe ingredients together and store in an airtight container.

To use, mix 2 tablespoons of the dry mixture with one egg yolk or one tablespoon of whole cow's milk or heavy cream or yogurt or coconut milk or wheatgerm oil.

Add 10 drops of essential oils that are beneficial for mature skin like geranium, clary sage, and lavender essential oils.

Apply the mixture as you massage it over the entire body and let it dry.

Rinse it off with warm water.

Moisturize the skin.

***

6. Pre-maturely Aging Skin Ubtan Recipe

Mix all the dry bridal ubtan recipe ingredients together and store in an airtight container.

To use, mix 2 tablespoons of the dry mixture with one egg yolk or one tablespoon of whole cow's milk or heavy cream or yogurt or coconut milk or wheatgerm oil.

Add 10 drops of essential oils that are beneficial for pre-maturely aging skin include patchouli, clary sage, rose, lavender and geranium essential oils.

Apply the mixture as you massage it over the entire body and let it dry.

Rinse it off with warm water.

Moisturize the skin.

***

7. Cellulite Ubtan Recipe

Mix all the dry bridal ubtan recipe ingredients together and store in an airtight container.

To use, mix 2 tablespoons of the dry mixture with one egg yolk or one tablespoon of whole cow's milk or heavy cream or yogurt or coconut milk or wheatgerm oil.

Add 10 drops of essential oils that are beneficial for cellulite like geranium, rosemary, sweet orange, lemon, lemongrass, grapefruit, juniper, and rosewood essential oils.

Apply the mixture as you massage it over the entire body and let it dry.

Rinse it off with warm water.

Moisturize the skin.

*****

6
Characteristics Of Essential Oils That Can Be Used To Make Ubtan Powders

Choose the aromatherapy essential oils to use depending on the effects you want the bath bomb to have. For example:

Clary Sage Essential Oil has an herbaceous scent. It can help relieve stress related tension, reduce irritability and help one relax. It is also used for the management of mature and acne prone skin. Do not use it during pregnancy or if you are drinking alcohol or driving or if you have endometriosis, ovarian cysts, uterine cysts, breast cancer or you are at high risk for developing breast cancer as it may have an "estrogen-like" effect on the body.

Eucalyptus essential oil has an invigorating scent. It can help relieve stress related mental tension and mental exhaustion. It is also used in the management of joint aches and pains. Do not use eucalyptus essential oil if you have epilepsy, high blood pressure or apply it near a baby's nostrils.

Geranium Essential Oil has a fresh, minty rose scent. It can help relieve nervous tension and anxiety. It is also used in the management of eczema, cellulite as well as mature skin. Avoid using it in pregnancy.

Grapefruit essential oil has a refreshing, bitter-sweet scent. It can help relieve tension and release repressed emotions. It is also used in the management of cellulite.

Lavender essential oil has a soothing, floral scent. It can help one relax and relieve stress related tension, sleeplessness, anxiety and depression. It is also used in the management of acne, eczema and dry skin conditions. Do not use lavender essential oil in pregnancy, if you are breastfeeding, on young children as it may cause breast development in young boys and girls. Avoid it if you have low blood pressure as you may feel drowsy after using it.

Lemon essential oil has an clarifying fresh scent. It can help relieve mental tension, alleviate mental fatigue and increase concentration. It is also used in the management of acne and post acne dark skin spots. Do not use it if skin will be exposed to sunlight or UV rays in the next 12-24 hours. Do not use it if you have low blood pressure or you are allergic to lemons.

Lemongrass essential oil has a vitalizing, lemony scent. It can help relieve tension and muscle aches. It is also used in the management of acne. Do not use it if skin will be exposed to sunlight or UV rays in the next 12-24 hours.

Roman chamomile essential oil has a sweet and fruity scent. It can help relieve stress related tension headaches. It is also used in the management of eczema, psoriasis and dry skin conditions. Avoid using it in pregnancy and if you are allergic to ragweed.

Spearmint essential oil has a gently-energizing minty scent. It can help relieve mental tension and exhaustion. It is also used in the management of nausea.

Rosemary Essential Oil has an uplifting and stimulating scent. It can help relieve mental exhaustion and feeling rundown. It is also used in the management of eczema, muscle aches and joint pains. Do not use rosemary essential oil if you are pregnant or have epilepsy or high blood pressure. Avoid using it if you have a fever or you want to sleep and in children under 5 years.

Sweet orange essential oil has a cheeringly, refreshing scent. It can help mange stress related tension. It is also used in the management of cellulite and common colds. Do not use it if skin will be exposed to sunlight or UV rays in the next 12-24 hours.

Peppermint essential oil has a head-clearing, refreshing scent. It can help relieve tension and fatigue. It is also used to manage flatulence. Do not use peppermint essential oil in pregnancy, if breastfeeding, on children less than 5 years, if you have epilepsy or irregular heart beats or cardiac fibrillation or high blood pressure and before using a sun bed or going to hot humid places.

Tea tree essential oil has a purifying almost medicinal scent. It can help relieve tension and fatigue. It is also been used in the management of acne and athlete's foot.

Ylang ylang Essential Oil has a fragrantly floral scent. It can help relieve anxiety, tension and help one relax. It is also used as an aphrodisiac and in the management of dry skin conditions. Do not use ylang ylang essential oil if you have low blood pressure or sensitive, damaged skin.

* * * * *

About The Author

Dr. Miriam Kinai is a medical doctor and a certified aromatherapist.

You can visit her blog at
http://www.TheBestSellingEbooks.blogspot.com/

or follow her on twitter at http://twitter.com/AlmasiHealth

Email enquiries to drkinai@yahoo.com with BOOKS as your subject.

Other Books By Dr Miriam Kinai

How to Make Natural Skincare Products 1

How to Make Natural Skincare Products volume 1 teaches you how to make:

1. Bath bombs

2. Bath melts

3. Bath salts

4. Bath teas

5. Body butters

6. Body lotions

7. Body scrubs

8. Healing balms

9. Herb infused oils

10. Natural soap

*****

Aromatherapy Course

Aromatherapy Course uses clear explanations and numerous recipes to teach you how to use essential oils to improve you physical, mental and emotional well being.

This home-study course covers the profiles of 30 essential and carrier oils as well as the safety precautions and you need to keep in mind when using them.

Each of the 10 lessons in this self paced course ends with practical exercises on how to use these healing aromatherapy oils so that persons with no previous training in aromatherapy can begin utilizing their healing benefits.

You will learn:

* How to blend essential oils

* How to dilute essential oils with carrier oils

* How to administer essential oils

* The therapeutic uses of essential oils like clary sage, eucalyptus, geranium, grapefruit, lavender, lemon, lemongrass, marjoram, orange (sweet), patchouli, peppermint, Roman chamomile, rose, rosemary, sandalwood, spearmint, tea tree and ylang ylang.

* * * * *

Medical Aromatherapy for Healthcare Professionals

Medical Aromatherapy for Healthcare Professionals teaches you how to use essential oils to treat physical diseases and emotional disorders.

The author's experience as a medical doctor and clinical aromatherapy practitioner have enabled her to write a highly informative guide for those who want to utilize the healing benefits of these natural plant essences.

You will discover how to use essential oils to:

* Treat skin diseases like acne, eczema and psoriasis

* Treat other physical diseases like high blood pressure, arthritis, coughs and colds

* Manage mental and emotional conditions like anxiety, depression, anger and stress

* Relieve the symptoms of menopause and premenstrual tension

* Lessen insomnia and impotence

Medical Aromatherapy for Healthcare Professionals is therefore an essential resource for holistic healthcare practitioners like massage therapists, naturopaths and herbalists.

It is also a useful resource for conventional medicine healthcare providers like physicians and nurses who want to begin practicing integrative medicine and for patients who want to improve their health naturally by using aromatherapy oils.

*****

Christian Life Coaching

Christian Life Coaching teaches you the Biblical principles to help you lead a more successful life. Topics covered include:

* Christian anger management

* Christian conflict resolution strategies

* Christian goal setting

* Christian personal finance

* Christian stress management

* Christian marital stress management

* How to deal with depression Biblically

* How to assert yourself

* How to stop being a people pleaser

* How to cure fear

* How to resist temptation

* How to love yourself

* * * * *

Dark Skin Dermatology Color Atlas

Dark Skin Dermatology Color Atlas is filled with clear explanations and color photos of skin, hair, and nail diseases affecting people with skin of color or Fitzpatrick skin types IV, V, and VI.

Topics covered include Acne Vulgaris, Alopecia Areata, Anal Warts, Angioedema, Aphthous Ulcers, Atopic Dermatitis, Blastomycosis, Blister Beetle Dermatitis or Nairobi Fly Dermatitis, Cellulitis, Chronic Ulcers, Confetti Hypopigmentation, Cutaneous T Cell Lymphoma, Cutaneous Tuberculosis, Dermatitis Artefacta, Erythema Nodosum, Exfoliative Erythroderma, Gianotti Crosti Syndrome, Hand Dermatitis , Hemangioma, Herpes Zoster, Ichthyosis, Ingrown Toenails, Irritant Contact Dermatitis, Kaposi Sarcoma, Keloids, Keratoderma Blenorrhagica, Klippel Trenaunay Weber Syndrome, Leishmaniasis, Leprosy, Leukonychia, Lichen Nitidus, Lichen Planus, Lichenoid Drug Eruption, Linear Epidermal Nevus, Linear IgA Dermatosis (LAD), Lipodermatosclerosis, Lymphangioma Circumscriptum, Miliaria, Molluscum Contagiosum, Neurofibromatosis, Nickel Dermatitis, Onychomadesis, Onychomycosis, Palmoplantar Eccrine Hidradenitis, Papular Pruritic Eruption (PPE), Paronychia, Pellagra, Pemphigus Foliaceous, Pemphigus Vulgaris, Piebaldism, Pityriasis Rosea, Pityriasis Rubra Pilaris, Plantar Hyperkeratosis, Plantar Warts, Poikiloderma, Postinflammatory Hyperpigmentation and Hypopigmentation, Post Topical Steroids Hypopigmentation, Psoriasis, Pyogenic Granuloma or Lobular Capillary Hemangioma, Scabies, Seborrheic Dermatitis, Steven Johnson Syndrome (SJS) and Toxic Epidermal Necrolysis (TEN), Sunburn, Systemic Sclerosis, Tinea Capitis, Tinea Pedis, Tinea Versicolor, Traction Alopecia, Urticaria, Vasculitis, Vitiligo, and Xanthelasma.

* * * * *

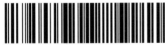

Made in the USA
San Bernardino, CA
29 April 2018